Michelle Finds a Voice

Sheila Hollins and Sarah Barnett,
illustrated by Denise Redmond

s Beyond Words

.ll/St George's Hospital Medical School
ɔN

First published in Great Britain 1997 by Gaskell and St George's
Hospital Medical School.

ISBN 1 901242 06 4

British Library Cataloguing-in-Publication Data

A catalogue record for this book is available from the British
Library.

Printed and bound in Great Britain by Acanthus Press Limited,
Wellington, Somerset TA21 8ST

Further information about the Books Beyond Words series
can be obtained from:

Royal College of Psychiatrists
17 Belgrave Square
London SW1X 8PG

Tel: 0171 235 2351
Fax: 0171 245 1231

Acknowledgements

We are grateful to many people who gave their time most generously to help us, in particular: Helen Allum, Dorothea Duncan, Peter Edwards, Nigel Hollins, Janet Larcher, Debbie Leach, Anthony Robertson.

Thanks also to the students on the General Education and Pre-Vocational Access Course, South Thames College.

We are grateful to **Communication Matters** for financial support for this project.

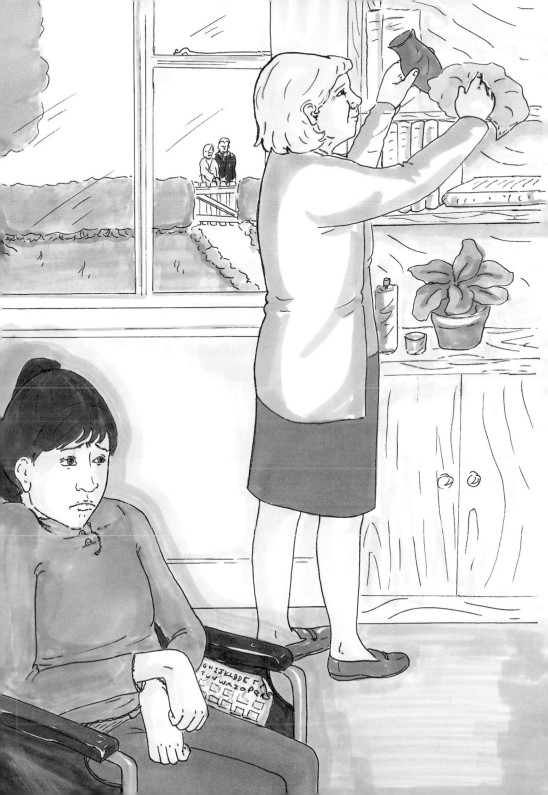

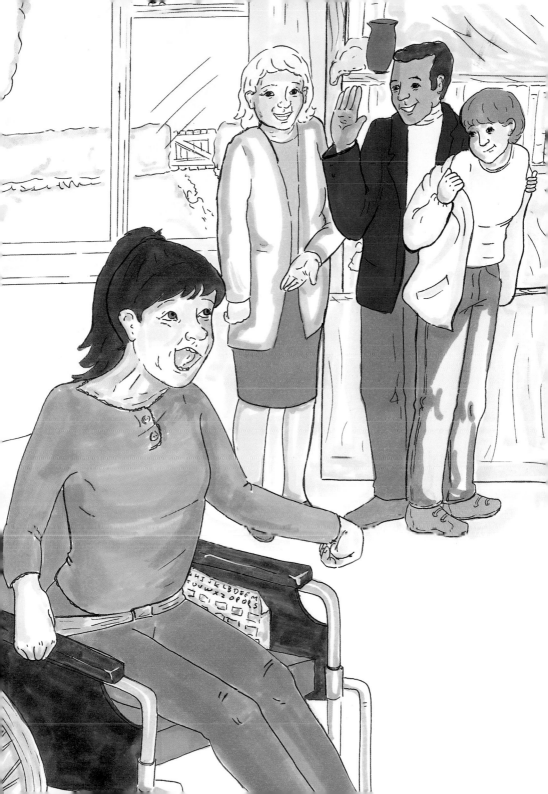

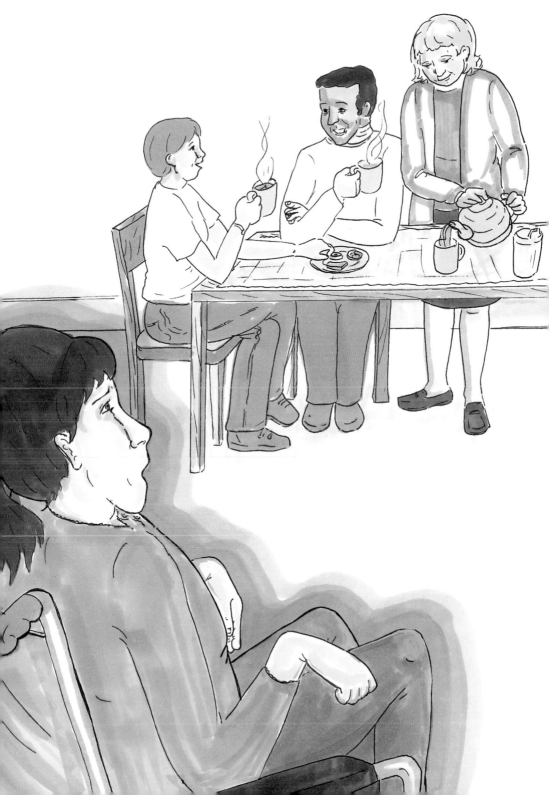

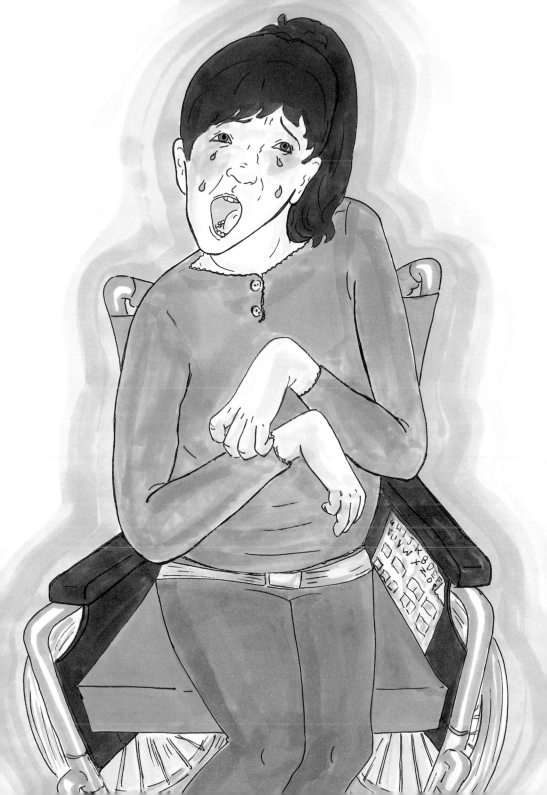

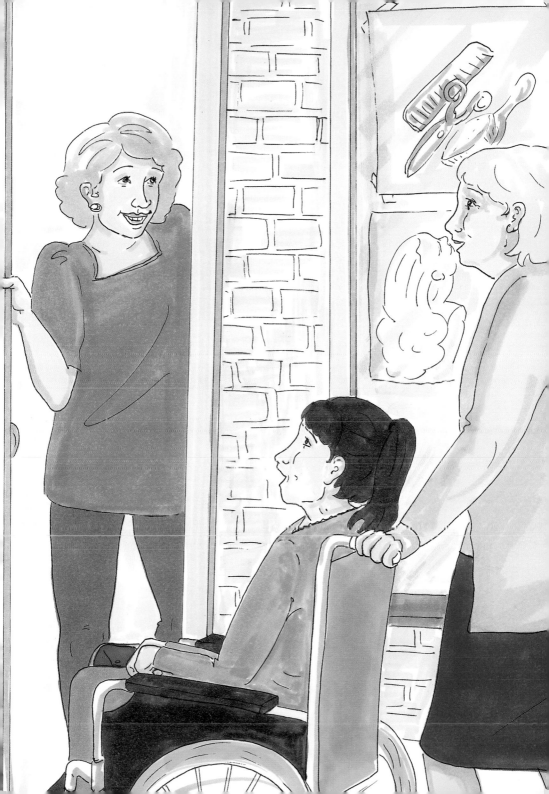

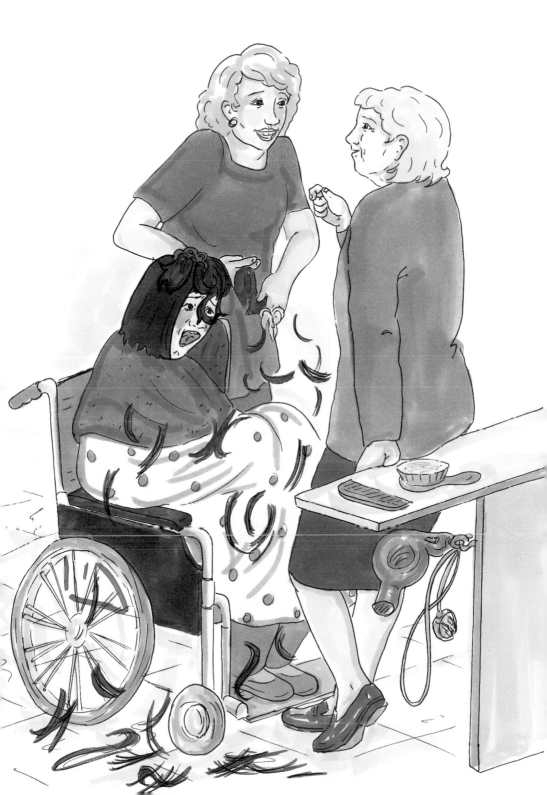

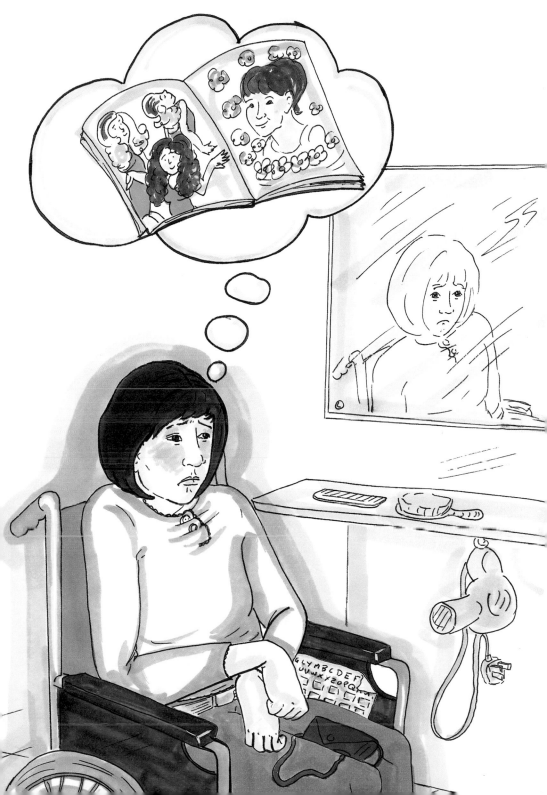

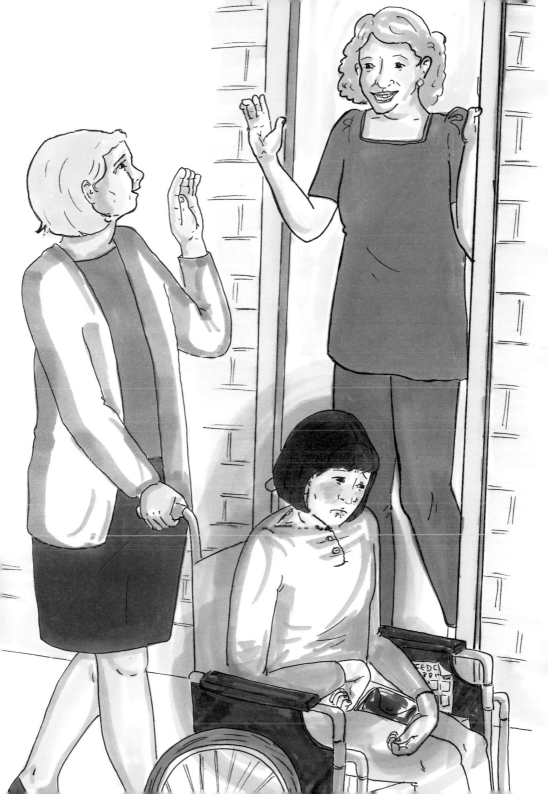

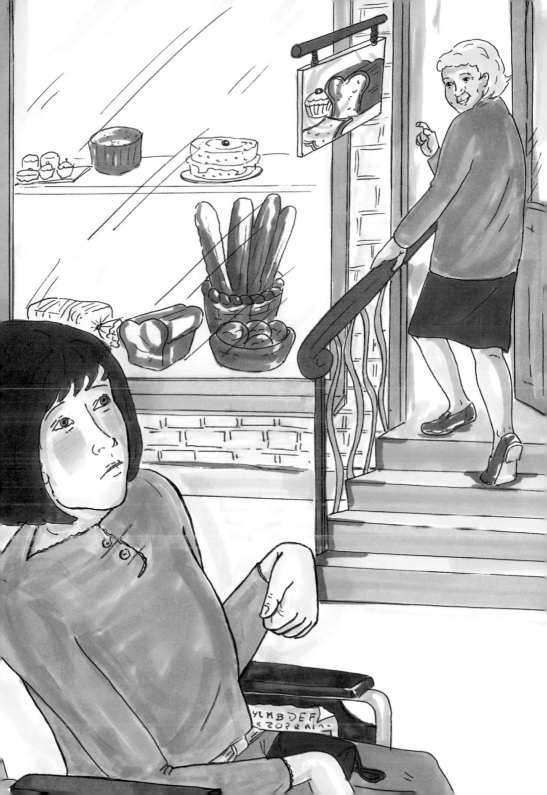

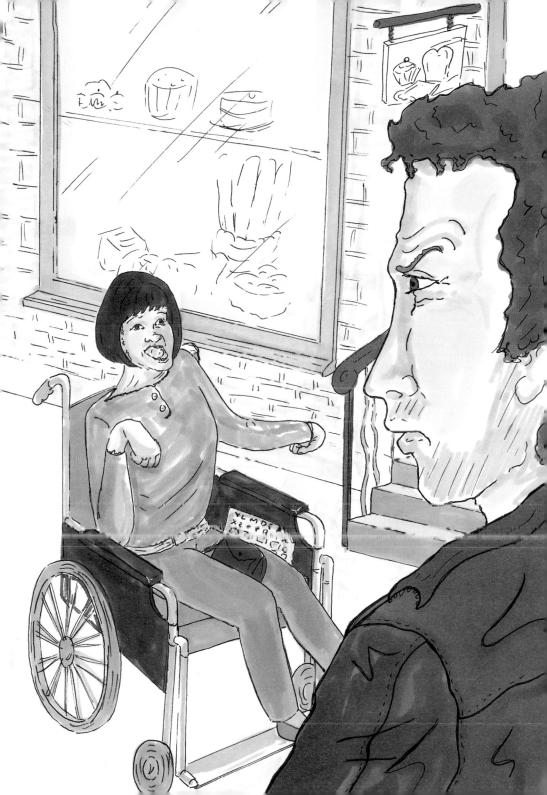

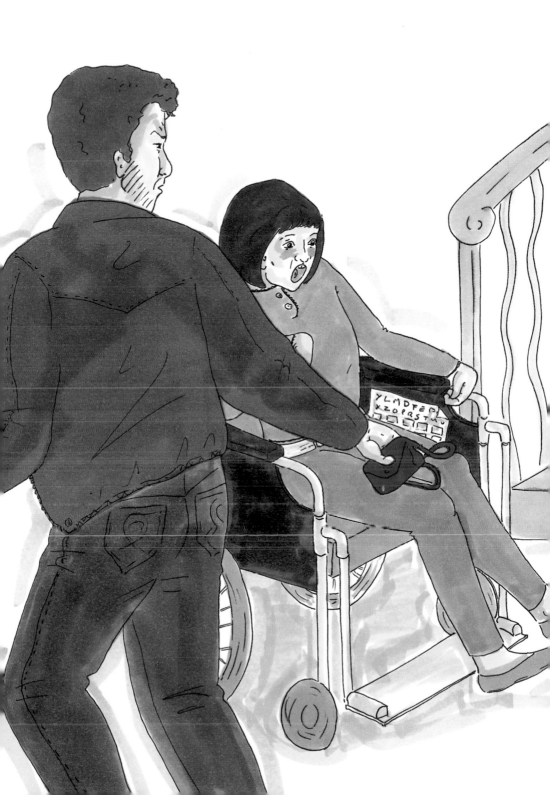

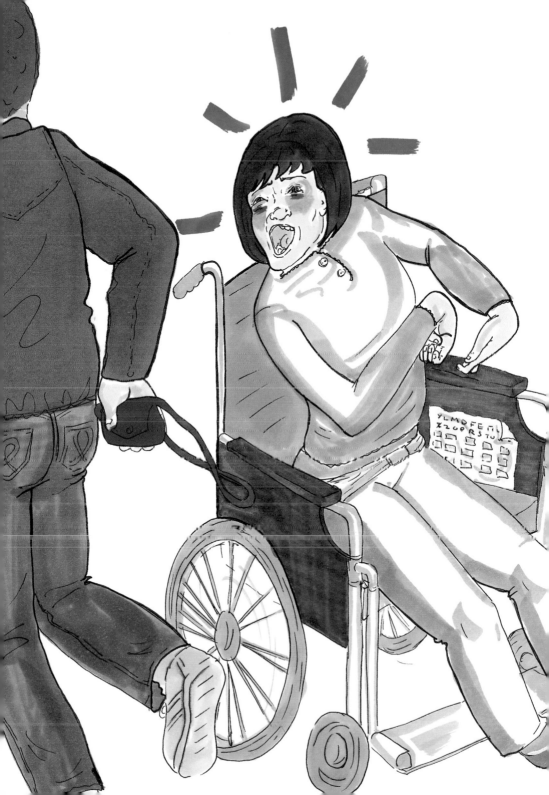

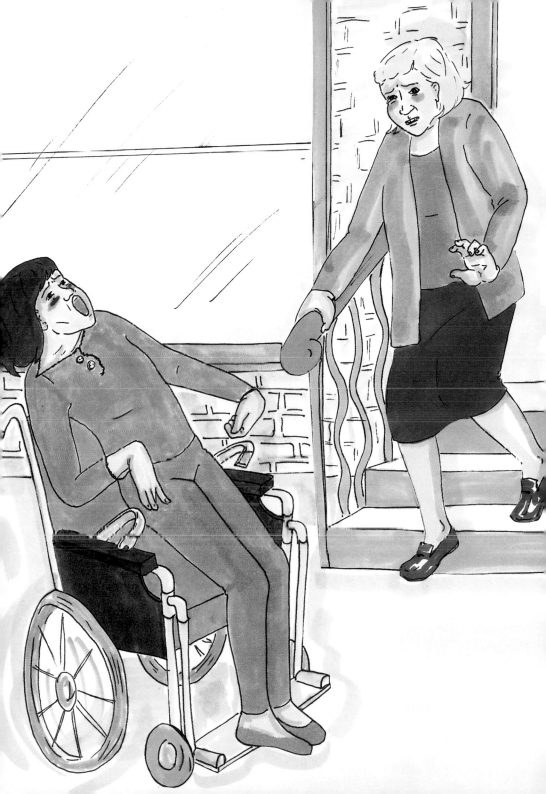

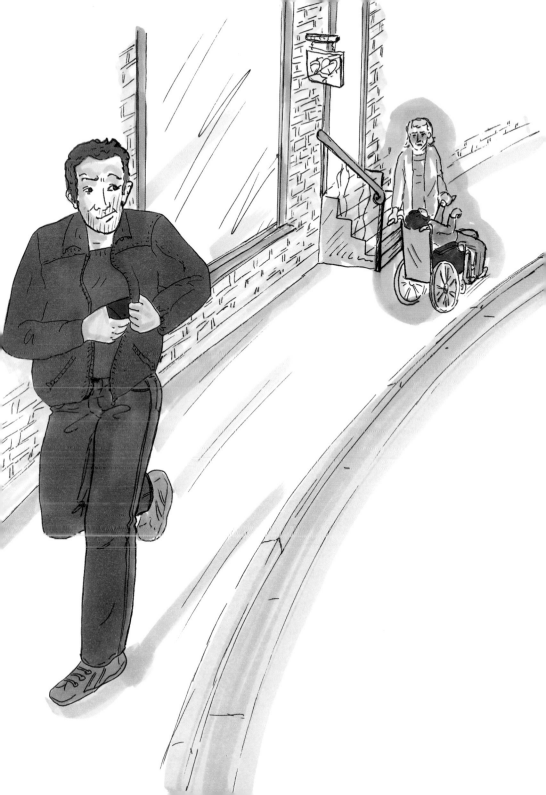

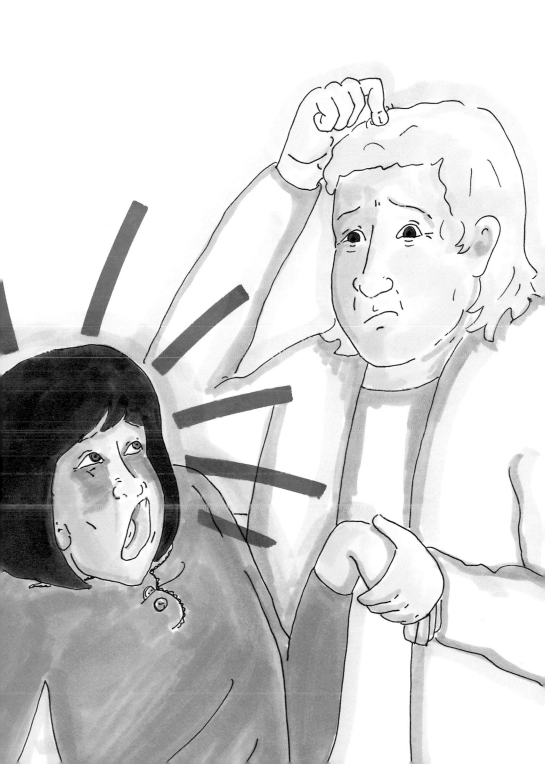

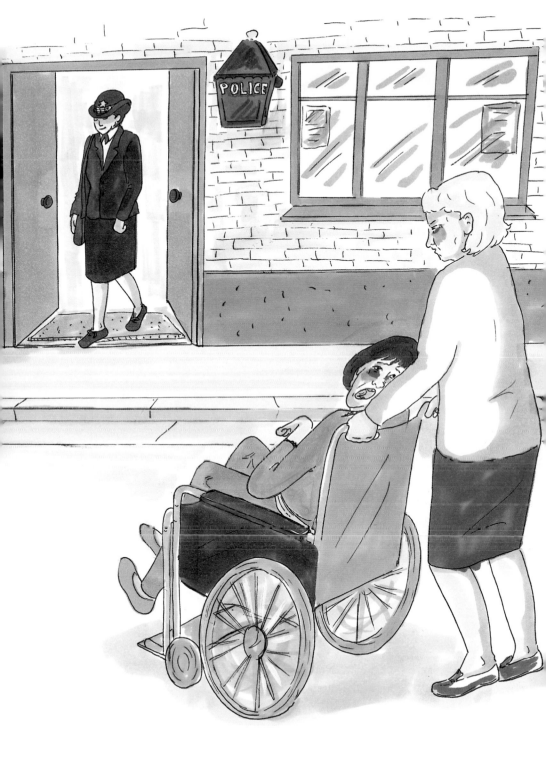

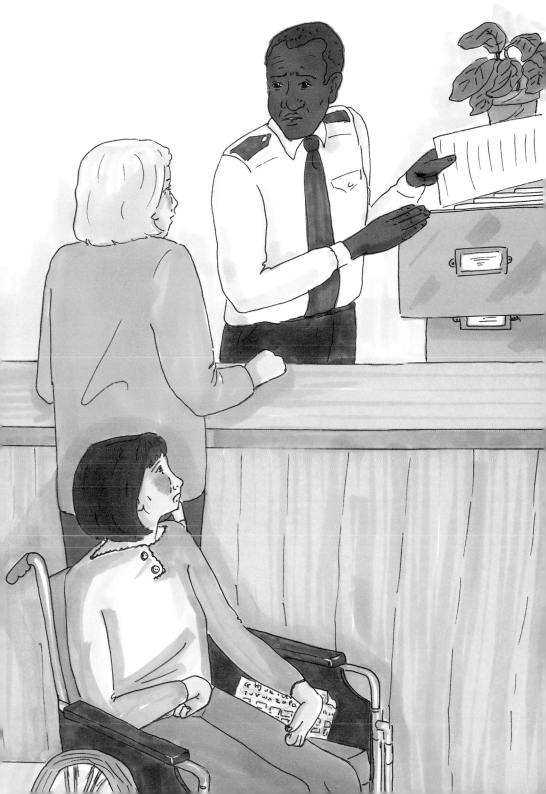

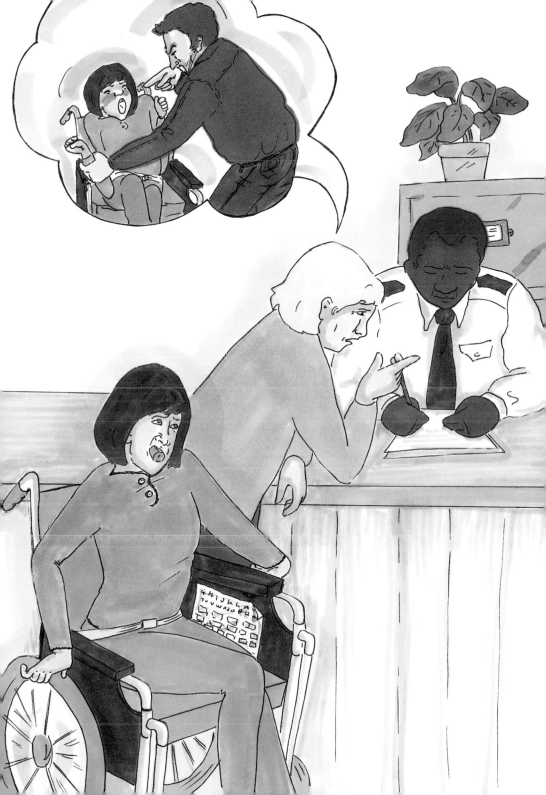

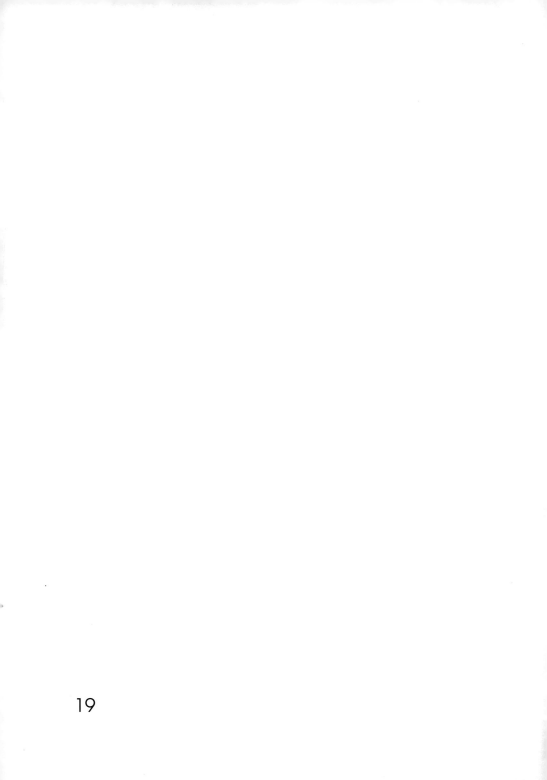

19

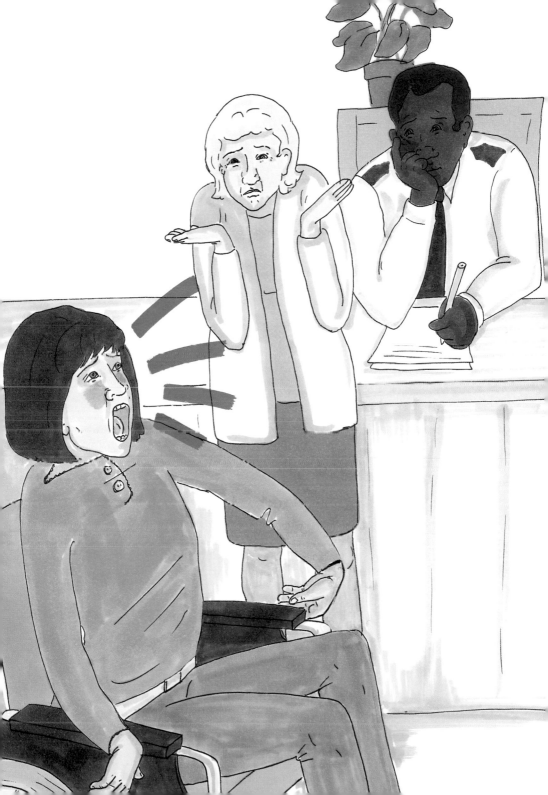

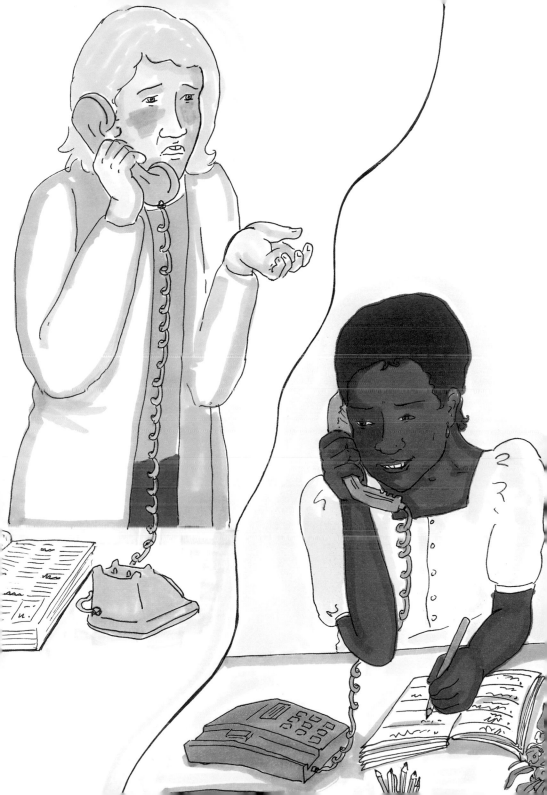

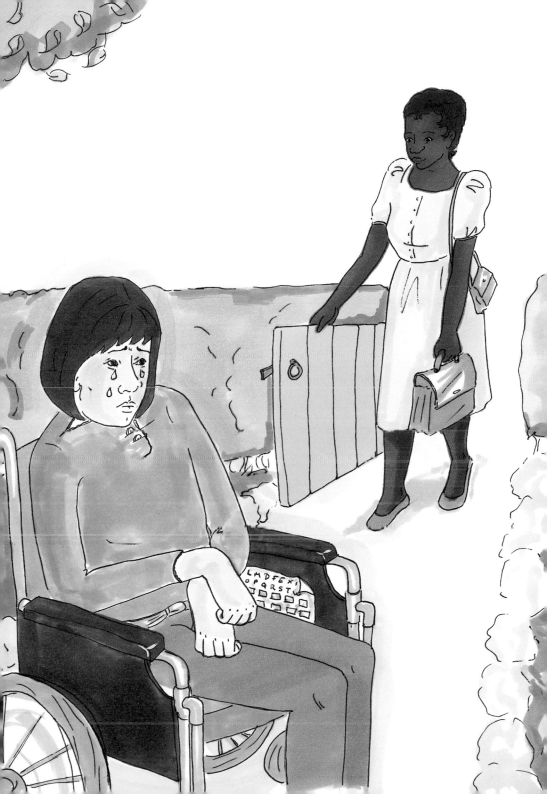

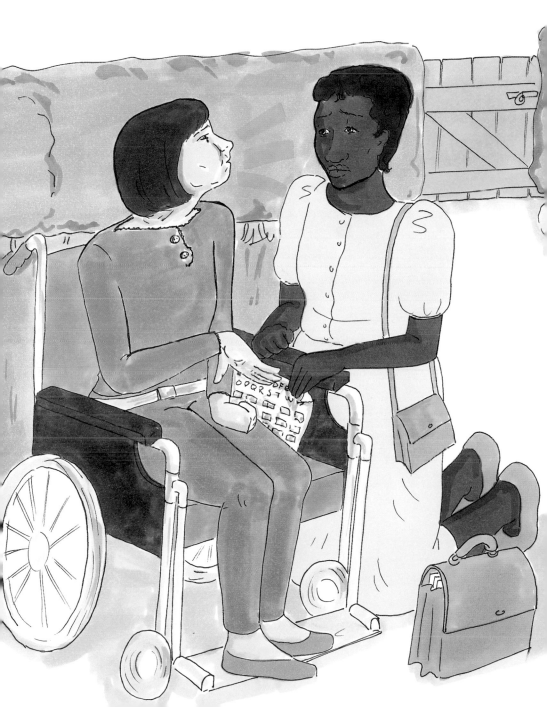

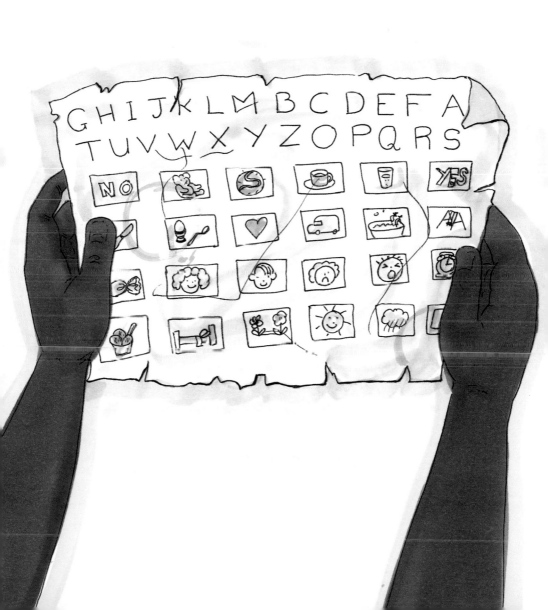

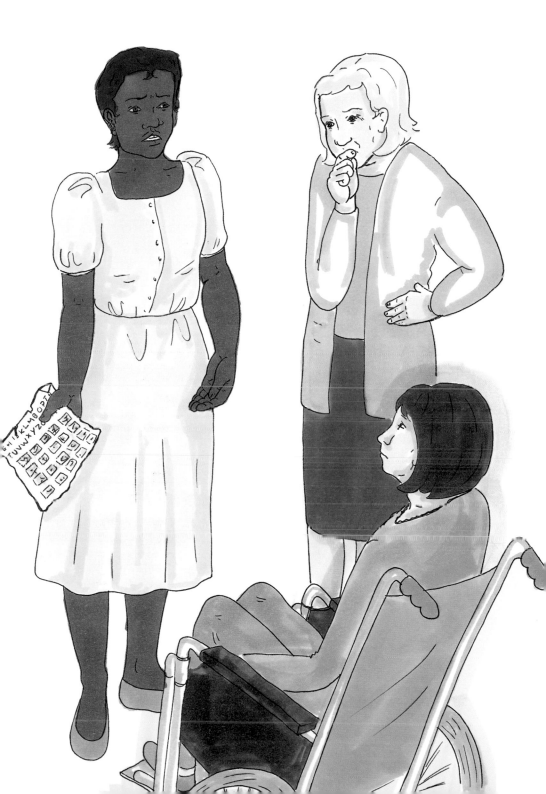

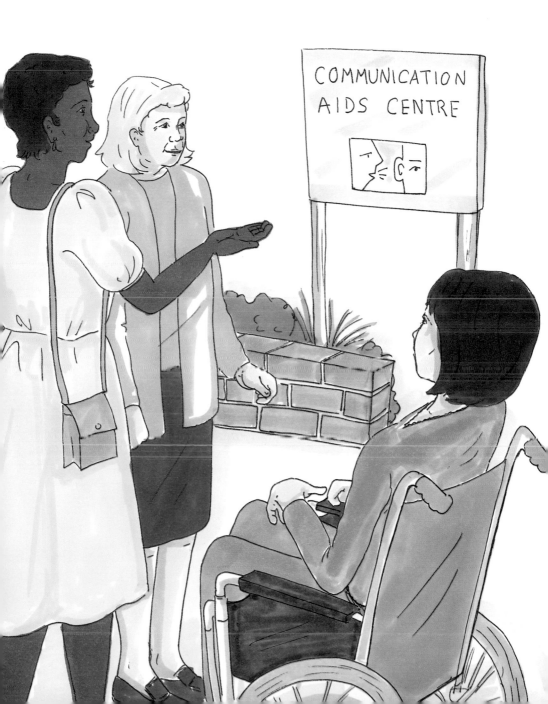

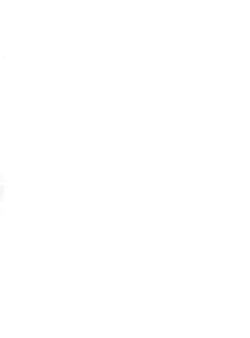

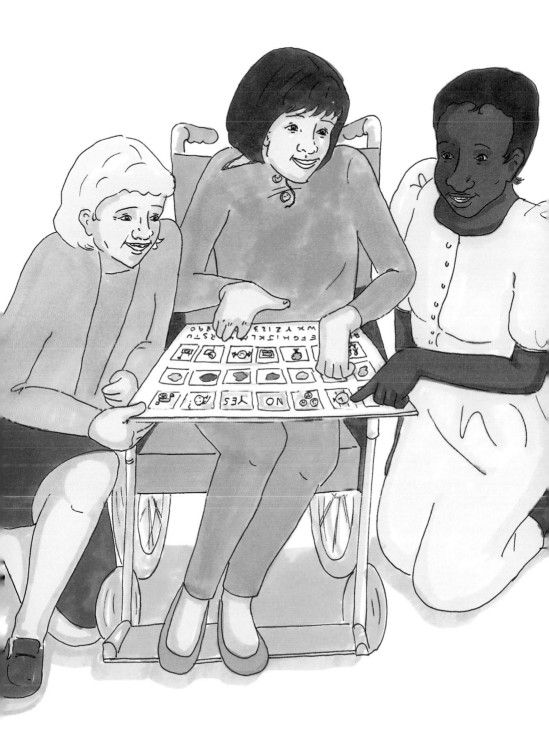

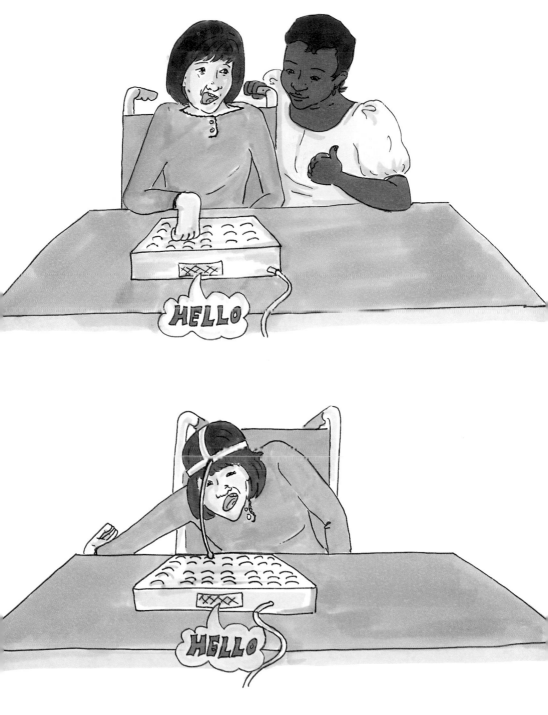

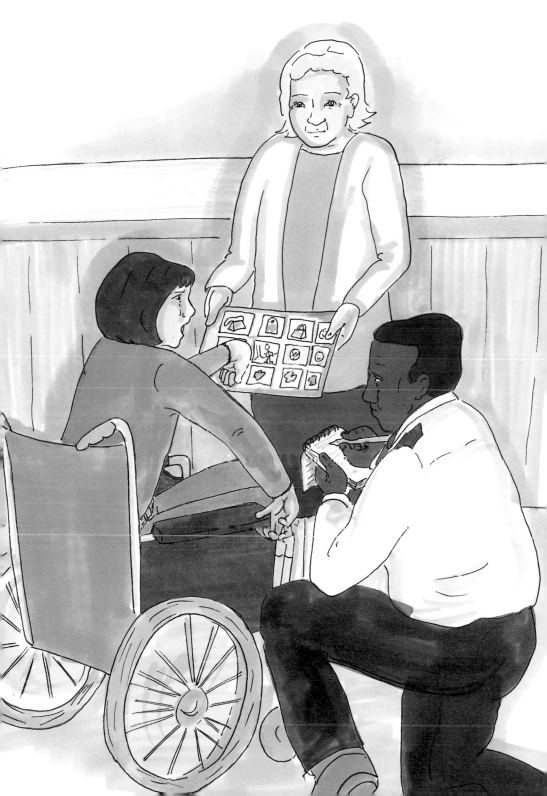

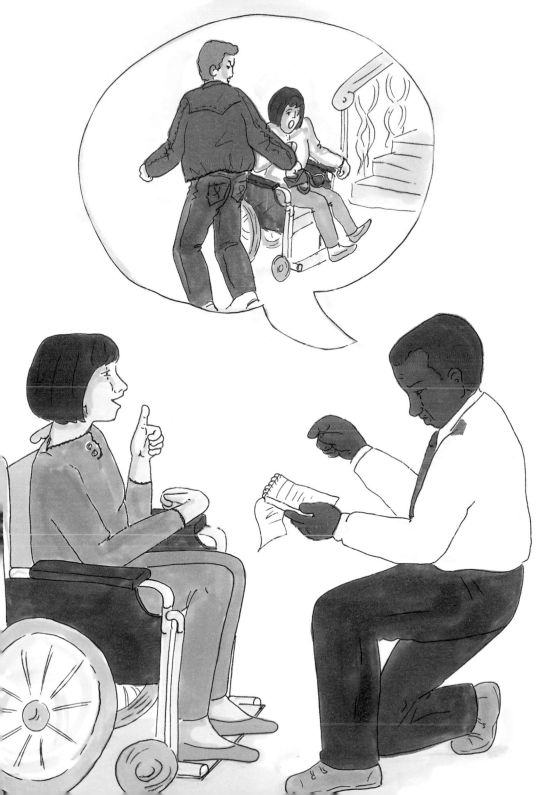

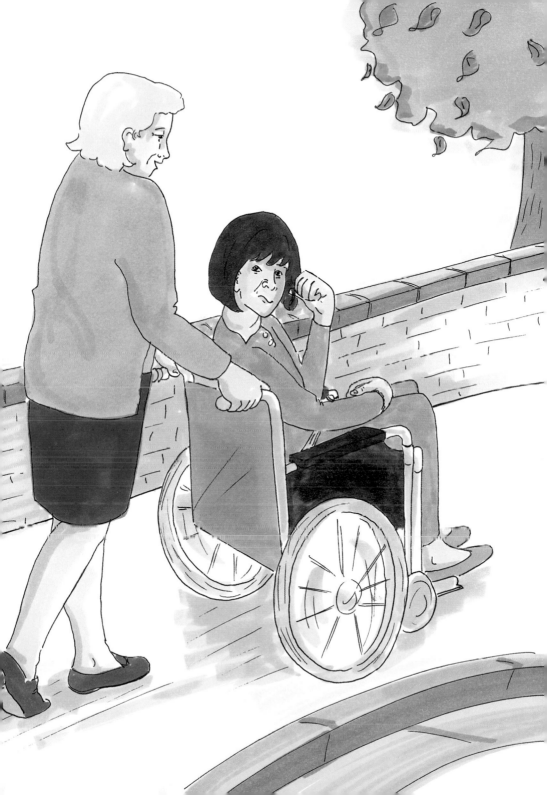

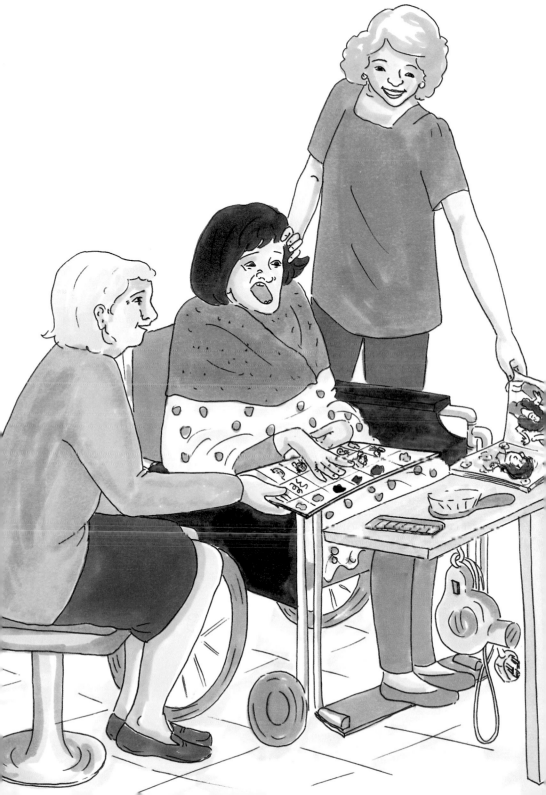

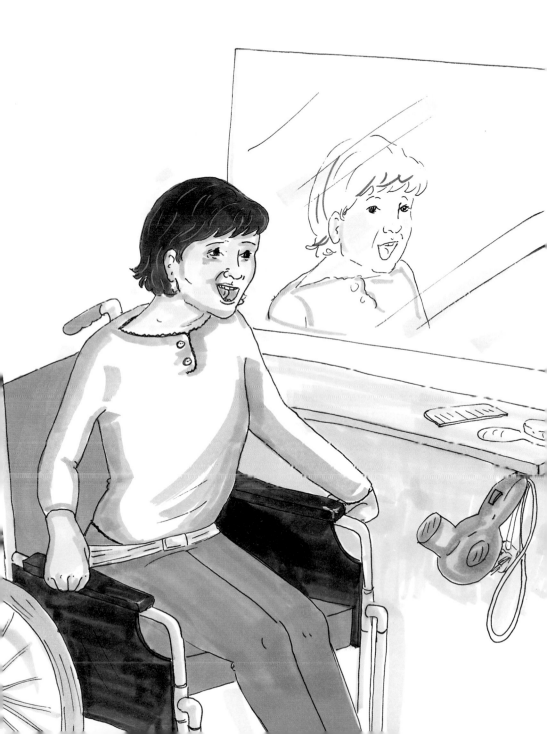

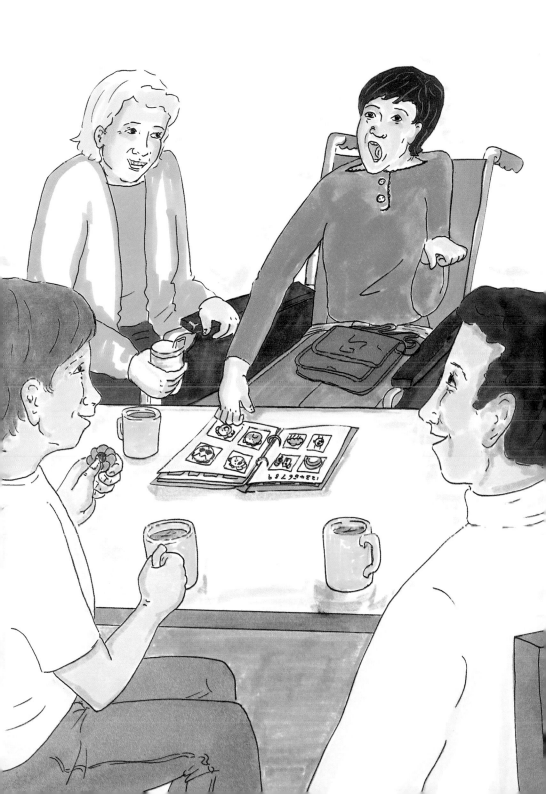

The following words are provided for readers or carers who want a ready-made story rather than to make up their own. ('Mum' could be a friend or carer).

Picture numbers

1. Michelle is sitting in her wheelchair. She can't walk. She can't talk. Mum is dusting the shelf.
2. Michelle's friends, Tom and Lynne, have arrived.
3. Lynne, Mum and Tom are talking together. They are ignoring Michelle.
4. Michelle feels upset and left out.
5. Mum is taking Michelle down town to the hairdresser. The hairdresser is called Jo.
6. Michelle is having her hair cut. Jo is talking to Mum.
7. Michelle looks at her new hairstyle in the mirror. She doesn't like it. She wanted a different style. She liked the hairstyle in the magazine.
8. Mum says goodbye to Jo. Michelle looks fed up.
9. Mum goes into the bakers.
10. A man stops and looks at Michelle.
11. He steals her handbag.
12. Michelle screams for help.
13. Mum comes out. "What's the matter?"
14. Mum sees the man running away.
15. Mum asks what happened, and tries to calm Michelle down.
16. Mum and Michelle go the police station.

17. Mum talks to the policeman.

18. Mum says the man hurt Michelle and was rude to her.

19. Michelle tries to say "that's not what happened." Mum and the policeman don't understand.

20. Mum phones Ann. Ann is a speech and language therapist.

21. Michelle is crying – she's in the garden. Ann comes to see her.

22. Ann asks what's the matter.

23. Ann looks at her old communication chart. It has the wrong words on it.

24. Ann shows the chart to Mum.

25. Ann takes Mum and Michelle to the Communication Aids Centre.

26. Ann shows Mum and Michelle a better communication chart.

27. Michelle tries some different communication aids.

28. Michelle uses her new communication charts to explain to the policeman what really happened.

29. The policeman can understand now.

30. Mum takes Michelle back to the hairdresser.

31. This time Jo and Mum listen to what Michelle wants. Michelle uses her new chart. She explains how she wants her hair.

32. She likes her new hairstyle.

33. Her friends have come to visit again. Michelle finds it easier to join in with them now. She is telling them her news, using her new communication book.

Thinking about communication

Communication is the Essence of Human Life.

International Society of Augmentative and Alternative Communication
Mission Statement

We use communication to:

express needs and wants:	i.e. choice making but there is life beyond toilet and biscuit…
exchange information:	gossip, chat, give our news, express our worries, share our feelings, ask questions, discuss, argue…
develop close relationships:	can I sit next to you? would you like to come to tea?
conform to social politeness:	hello/bye; please/thanks; sorry…

Janice Light, 1988

We use our voices to speak but communicate with our whole body. To empower people with learning difficulties, we need to give them the signs and symbols vocabulary to introduce their own topics into the conversation – not just to make choices about their needs and wants.

People with learning difficulties need to communicate with each other and with the wider community, just as we all do – not just in timetabled communication sessions.

Research studies have proved that signing and/or using symbol systems may facilitate speech development.

Keyworker: "I don't use symbols with her any more, because she knows them."
Speech and language therapist: "How would you feel if we stopped using words with you, because you know them?"

An augmentative and alternative communication (AAC) system does not result in instant communication any more than providing a piano results in an instant musician.

It takes a long time for a person to become competent with an AAC system. For comparison, it is estimated that it takes 200 teaching hours before a foreign student is competent to carry out a basic conversation in English. However, it is estimated that AAC users are likely at best to get only 40 hours' input a year (Murphy *et al*, 1996).

A long-term support and development programme is essential, and the carer's implementation of the agreed programme is crucial to its success.

Light, J. (1988) Interaction involving individuals using augmentative and alternative communication systems: state of the art and future directions for research. *Augmentative and Alternative Communication*, **4**, 66–82.

Murphy, J., Marková, I., Collins, S. & Moodie, E. (1996) AAC systems: obstacles to effective use. *European Journal of Disorders of Communication*, **31**, 31–44.

Communication systems

Augmentative and alternative communication

For people with severe communication impairments, there are a number of different types of AAC systems which, alone or in combination, may help them:

- For people with reasonably good hand function, manual signing is an option. For example, simple gesture, sign systems, sign language, finger spelling.

- Some people show what they want to say by pointing to pictures, symbols or letters on a chart or in a book. There are many different symbol systems available, suitable for users at different ages and stages.

- Nowadays there is also a range of microelectronic technology – from simple to complex – which can increase independence. Voice Output Communication. Aids (VOCAs) give people a voice that can be heard. Computers can enable people to write, work, control their environment and communicate electronically with others throughout the world.

Symbol systems

Objects of Reference are used with people who have profound and multiple learning difficulties, and with people who have visual or dual sensory impairments. Such systems use real objects chosen to represent a particular activity. These may gradually become symbols. This can be done by reducing them in size, by using just part of the object, or by using a texture associated with the object.

Photographs, particularly of important people in a person's life, are often useful in communication charts and books.

Pictures, including commercially available picture stickers, or logos of favourite food items etc., are often useful in communication charts and books.

Picture Communication Symbols (PCSs) is an American symbol system, comprising 2000–3000 symbols. They are simple line drawings in black-on-white or in colour. They are fairly widely used in the UK, and computer software is available for easier creation of communication charts (Don Johnston).

Rebus Symbols were originally devised to help develop reading skills. There are about 4000 symbols, some are pictorial but others are more abstract and may be combined with letters. They are used in many day centres. They were one of the first systems available on computer software (Widgit).

Makaton Symbols were developed to correspond with the Makaton signing vocabularies. The core vocabulary contains many of the same symbols as Rebus. These symbols and line drawings of the Makaton signs are available on computer software (MUDP), but to create charts it is useful to use them in conjunction with the 'Gridmaker' programme (Widgit).

Other symbol systems include: Compic, PIC symbols, SIG symbols and Bliss symbols. Examples of some of the above symbol systems are shown in Figure 1.

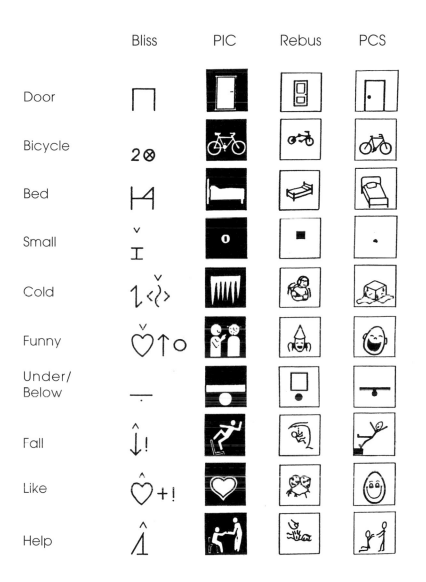

Figure 1. Symbol systems: Bliss, PIC, Rebus and PCS.

(Reproduced from *Augmentative and Alternative Communication: European Perspectives* (1996). Eds S. von Tetzchner and M. H. Jensen. London: Whurr Publishers.)

Signing systems

British Sign Language (BSL) is the language used by the deaf community in Britain. BSL is a naturally evolved language with its own structure, and so its grammar and word order is different from spoken and written English. Finger spelling is an intrinsic part of BSL. BSL signs can be adapted for single-handed use.

Signed English has been designed to mirror spoken English, and is taught to hearing-impaired children in some British schools, as a means of teaching English grammar. It is not a natural language. It's core vocabulary uses BSL signs with artificial signs added to mark the grammatical elements of English.

Cued Speech is a system for facilitating lip reading for people with hearing impairments. It uses eight hand shapes and four hand locations, combined with speech, to distinguish between sounds which look similar on the lips.

Paget Gorman signed speech is an artificial sign system, designed as a teaching tool for language-disordered children. It mirrors spoken English exactly, with one-to-one, sign-to-word correspondence. It uses complex and precise hand and finger positions.

Makaton was developed specifically for people with learning difficulties, and has been used in the majority of special schools and day centres in Britain and elsewhere since the 1970s. It is a vocabulary system, not a language. It is based on BSL signs although some have been modified to make them easier. Makaton signing is used to support spoken English, the key words are signed. It is possible to use one-handed signs in Makaton, and to do hand-over-hand signing for those with additional visual impairments.

Signalong is another a vocabulary system based on modified BSL signs. It too is for use with people with learning difficulties, but is much more recent and so less widespread. Many of the signs are similar to Makaton signs.

Resources

AAC Research Teams   01786 467645
Department of Psychology, University of Stirling, Stirling FK9 4LA
- Training videos and resources: Attitudes and Strategies Towards AAC, Talking to People with Severe Communication Difficulties
- AAC Skill Development Package

Able Net Inc.   01476 550391
Liberator Ltd, Whitegates, Swinstead, Lincolnshire NG33 4PA
- Communication aids/switches
- Assessment services

Call Centre   0131 667 1438
Communication Aids for Language and Learning, University of Edinburgh, 4 Buccleuch Place, Edinburgh EH8 9LW
- AAC Information, Research and Service Centre
- Series of videos and publications covering different aspects of the use of technology in helping people with special needs

The Disability Information Trust   01865 227600
Mary Marlborough Disability Centre, Nuffield Orthopaedic Centre, Headington, Oxford OX3 7LD
- Book: Communication and Access to Computer Technology, 1995
- Equipment for disabled people

Don Johnston Special Needs   01925 24164
18 Clarendon Court, Calver Road, Winwick Quay, Warrington WA2 8QP
- Software: PCS, Compic, DynaSyms, Blissymbols and Imaginart Boardmaker

Makaton Vocabulary Development Project
             01276 61390 (general) **01276 681368** (training)
31 Firwood Drive, Camberley, Surrey TU15 3QD
- Makaton signs and symbol software
- Makaton reference video

QED **01329 828444**
Ability House, 242 Gosport Road, Fareham, Hampshire PO16 0SS
- Switches and access to communication aids

The Symbols Working Group **0117 908 5000**
Phoenix NHS Trust, Brentree Hospital, Charlton Road, Westbury on Trym, Bristol BS10 6JH
- Resource pack on the use of symbols in every day situations: A Guide to Using Symbols

Widgit Software **01926 885303**
102 Radford Road, Leamington Spa CV31 1LF
- Software: Rebus symbols and picture collections, Gridmaker

Communication organisations: where to go for help and advice

Communication Matters is a national voluntary organisation concerned with the needs of people with severe communication difficulties. It is the UK branch of the International Society of Augmentative and Alternative Communication (ISAAC). Communication Matters can provide information and support with augmentative and alternative communication systems. These can maximise opportunities for disabled people, and enhance their lives. The organisation's members include AAC users, family members and carers of AAC users, as well as therapists, teachers, social workers, researchers, engineers and other professionals. It publishes an informative magazine three times a year. An annual conference is held each September at Lancaster University. For further information, contact:

Communication Matters **01254 673303** (answerphone)
c/o Lancashire School IT Centre, 103 Preston New Road, Blackburn BB2 6BJ

**Royal College of Speech and Language
Therapists** **0171 613 3855**
7 Bath Place, Rivington Street, London EC2A 3DA

Communication Aids Centres

CACs operate individually, the organisation and precise roles of each being different. The work of a CAC may include the assessment and treatment of clients with severe speech impairment, and the training and follow-up of clients in the use of communication aids/systems.

Always involve your local Speech and Language Therapist

Belfast CAC   **01232 669501**
Musgrave Park Hospital, Stockman's Lane, Belfast BT9 7JB

Bristol CAC   **0117 975 3947**
Speech and Language Therapy, Frenchay Hospital, Bristol BS16 1LE

Cardiff CAC   **01222 566281 (ext. 3708)**
Rookwood Hospital, Fairwater Road, Llandaf, Cardiff CF5 2YN

Charing Cross ACS   **0181 846 1057**
Charing Cross Hospital, Fulham Palace Road, London W6 8RF

Access to Communication and Technology   **0121 627 8235**
Oak Tree Lane Centre, Oak Tree Lane, Selly Oak, Birmingham B29 6JA

Communicate   **0191 233 1567**
The Lodge, Regional Rehabilitation Centre, Hunters Road, Newcastle upon Tyne NE3 1PH

Mary Marlborough Disability Centre   **01865 227600**
Nuffield Orthopaedic Centre, Windmill Road, Headington, Oxford OX3 7LD

Scottish Centre of Technology for the
Communication Impaired   **0141 201 6425/6**
Victoria Infirmary NHS Trust, Rutherglen Maternity Hospital, 120 Stonelaw Road, Rutherglen, Glasgow G73 2PG

Other relevant organisations

British Institute of Learning Disabilities   **01562 850251**
Wolverhampton Road, Kidderminster, Worcestershire DY10 3PP

Change   **0171 272 3526** (voice)
0171 561 9747 (minicom)
The National Deaf-Blind and Rubella Association, 11-13
Clifton Terrace, London N4 3SR

Disabled Living Foundation (DLF)   **0171 289 6111** (voice)
0171 432 8009 (minicom)
380-384 Harrow Road, London W9 2HU

MENCAP   **0171 454 0454**
MENCAP National Centre, 123 Golden Lane, London EC1Y 0RT

People First   **0171 713 6400**
207-215 Kings Cross Road, London WC1X 9DB

Royal Association for Disability and Rehabilitation (RADAR)
0171 250 3222 (voice)
0171 280 4119 (minicom)
Unit 12 City Forum, 250 City Road, London EC1V 8AF

Royal National Institute for the Deaf
0171 296 8000 (voice)
0171 296 8001 (minicom)
19-23 Featherstone Street, London EC17 8SL

Royal National Institute for the Blind   **0171 388 1266**
224 Great Portland Street, London W1N 6AA

Scope   **0171 636 5020**
12 Park Crescent, London W1N 4EQ
(From November 1997: 6-10 Market Road, London N7 0PN)

Sense   **0171 272 7774** (voice)
0171 272 9648 (minicom)
The National Deaf-Blind and Rubella Association, 11-13 Clifton
Terrace, London N4 3SR